Health Benefits
of
Apple Cider Vinegar

Improve Your Health and Wellness With Apple Cider Vinegar

RON KNESS

Published by:

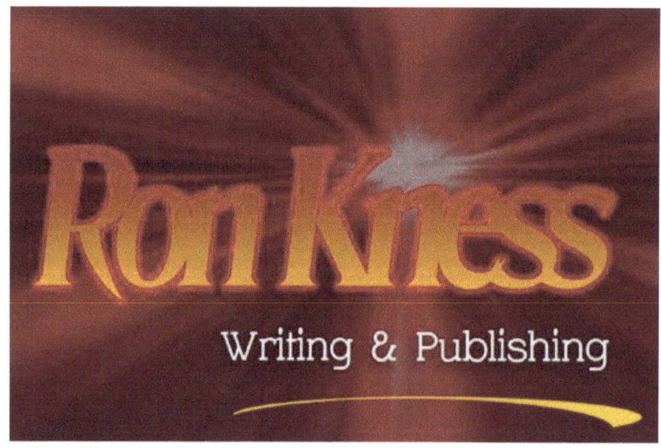

https://ronknesswriting.com

Ron Kness

Gold Canyon, AZ

United States of America

ISBN: 9781790396023

Apple Cider Vinegar Health Benefits

Disclaimer

We hope you enjoy reading this publication, however we do suggest you read our disclaimer. All the material written in this document is provided for informational purposes only and is general in nature.

Every person is a unique individual and what has worked for some or even many may not work for you. Any information perceived as advice must be considered in light of your own particular set of circumstances.

The author or person sharing this information does not assume any responsibility for the accuracy or outcome of your use of the content.

Every attempt has been made to provide well researched and up to date content at the time of writing. Now all the legalities have been taken care of, please enjoy the content.

See your healthcare professional before starting any diet, health or exercise program!

Introduction

Apple cider vinegar (ACV) is a remedial product that punches far above its weight in terms of efficacy versus cost and availability. It is readily available, cheaply, even at the supermarket. For human health, dosages are small – for most ailments a few teaspoons a day.

Before the advent of modern pharmacy, ACV was a health tonic and remedy in many households. Big pharma doesn't like it. It is too cheaply made and too ubiquitous to patent, so it holds no value for them.

Hordes of users attest to its ability to ease symptoms for many conditions. A great many use it as a morning tonic, to prevent the onset of many ailments and their symptoms.

This eBook explains what is known about how it works and what type of ACV you need to make sure it does.

There are chapters on specific conditions and how apple cider vinegar can help control the condition and alleviate the symptoms. Many will be interested in reading how to use ACV to control blood sugar levels and to assist with weight loss.

Apple Cider Vinegar and Our Acid and Alkaline Levels

Foods such as alcohol, sugar and other carbohydrates are some of the foods that cause increased acid levels in the body. Taking raw, unfiltered and unpasteurized apple cider vinegar before meals will help counteract this.

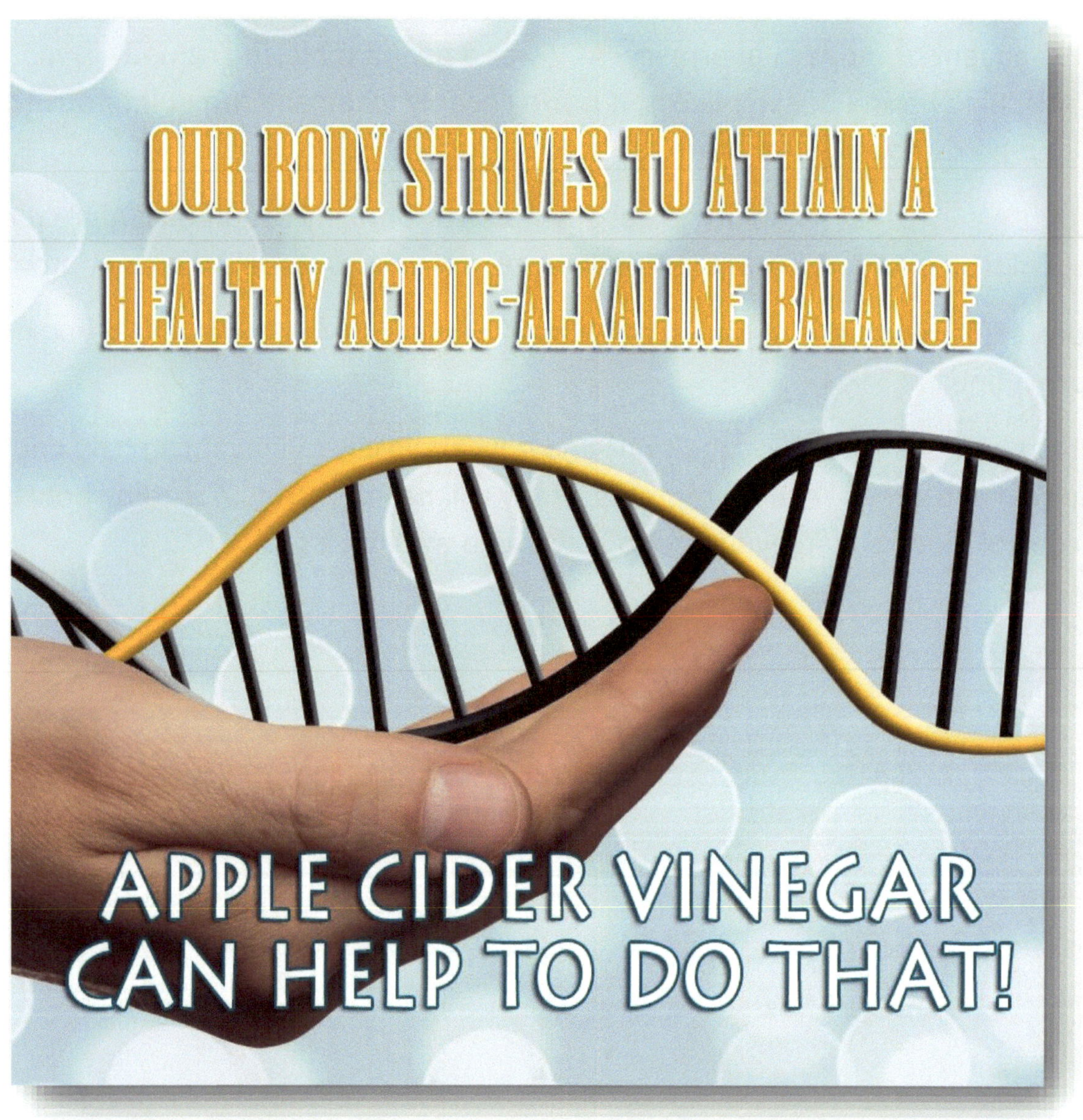

Lemons and raw unfiltered apple cider vinegar are both naturally acidic. However, because of the way they are metabolized when consumed, they become alkaline forming in the body.

Research has shown that our bodies strive to attain a healthy acidic-alkaline balance, although the majority of us tend to be more acidic than alkaline.

Opinions differ on the ideal health balance. A 60/40 alkaline-acid ratio is recommended by some advocates, while others suggest an 80/20 alkaline-acid ratio is more appropriate.

It is important to note that in a pH 'balanced' body, different parts of the body have different alkaline/acid ratios. For example, the pH of a healthy vagina may differ from the pH of the gut, even in the same person.

It is generally realized that our modern diet, with its heavy inclusion of simple carbohydrates, causes an overall acidification of our bodies, which provides an environment that allows non-beneficial microbes to thrive and multiply, to the detriment of our health and wellbeing. High acid levels in the body depletes energy and increases the risk of infection.

As well as keeping pathogens at bay, when the body is kept more alkaline, the increased energy level enables the body to more effectively fight off illness and disease. For most people, the first move towards improved health is ensuring the body becomes more alkaline.

Lifelong Benefits

It has been found that a high alkaline producing diet such as fruit and vegetables, and apple cider vinegar helps decrease the calorie burning muscle mass that is lost as we age.

A recent study of older adults found that those whose diets consisted of food that metabolized into alkaline residues had retained more muscle mass. The conclusion was that in some cases the outcome was almost enough to counteract the 4.4 pounds of lean tissue that is typically lost each decade as we age.

Apple Cider Vinegar Helps Neutralize Stomach Acid

It is believed that apple cider vinegar helps to balance the pH in the stomach by neutralizing the acid. This effectually helps eliminate heartburn and acid reflux. When stomach acid leaks back into the esophagus, it results in an unpleasant burning feeling in the chest or throat known as heartburn or acid reflux.

When the food in the stomach is in a milder acidic environment it will still be digested efficiently. However, with less acid there will be fewer problems with the esophagus, and less chance of acid reflux or heartburn.

A recent survey conducted by the Earth Clinic website nominated apple cider vinegar as the most popular and best home remedy to relieve symptoms of heartburn and acid reflux.

A dose of 10-15 mls (2 – 3 teaspoons) of apple cider vinegar in a glass of water before meals or whenever an episode of heartburn or reflux is experienced is recommended. If the taste of the vinegar is a deterrent add the dose to a glass of fruit juice and the taste will be almost unnoticeable.

It will also benefit general health to add apple cider vinegar to your cooking or use as a salad dressing.

Apple Cider Vinegar With the "Mother"

Unrefined, unfiltered and unpasteurized apple cider vinegar is considered to have the most health benefits. Quality vinegar like this contains what is known as the mother.

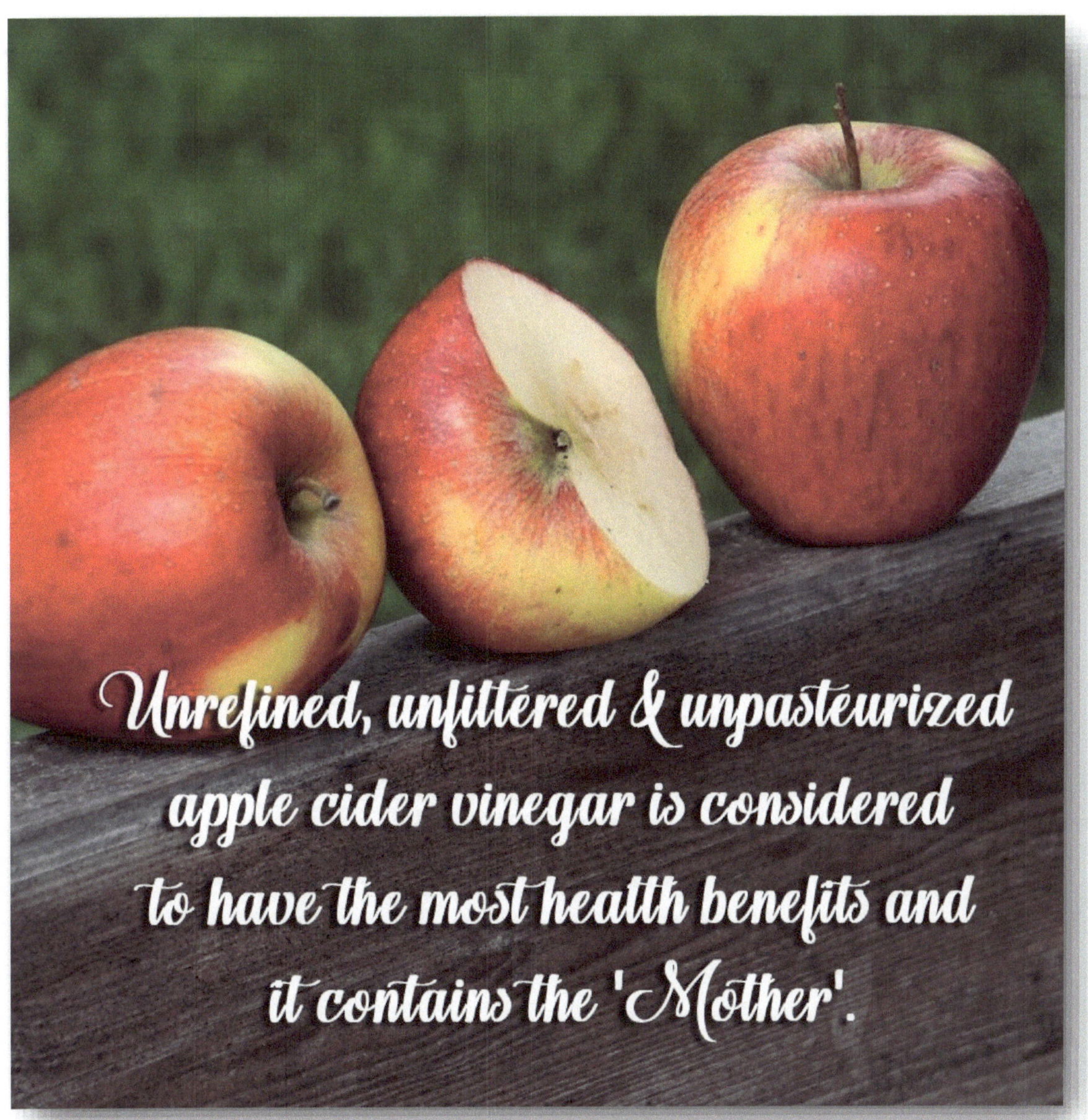

The appearance is dark brown with strands resembling cobwebs. As it is unfiltered the product may appear cloudy or contain some sediment at the bottom of the container.

The mother itself is a rich, natural, health boosting protein. The gut- friendly bacteria, enzymes and acetic acid of the mother help keep the digestive system working efficiently. It has a neutralizing effect on stomach acid and is known to be very effective in fighting harmful bacteria.

The Health Benefits of Unpasteurized Apple Cider Vinegar

The healing restorative properties that are formed through the fermentation process of apple cider vinegar remain intact when the vinegar is raw, unfiltered, unpasteurized and contains the live mother.

This ability is considered by some to be the most important property of this versatile health food. The wide range of health problems that are helped by the use of this very popular apple cider vinegar is indeed amazing.

The raw unpasteurized apple cider vinegar contains pectin, a prebiotic which is a great aid to digestive disorders.

Increasing evidence implicates an imbalance in gut flora (where harmful bacteria exist in unnatural amounts) as causing and contributing to a large range of health problems, from relatively minor to very serious. Imbalance in the body is believed to be the cause of numerous problems affecting the health of many people.

The inclusion of unpasteurized apple cider vinegar in the diet has been proven to have the ability to bring balance back to the body. The beneficial effects of apple cider vinegar in helping neutralize these pathogens cannot be over-emphasized.

Studies have found unpasteurized apple cider vinegar containing the mother helps lower blood sugar levels and has the ability to aid the recovery process if you are sick.

The Process of Making Apple Cider Vinegar

Two steps are involved in the making of apple cider vinegar. The process begins with yeast being added to apple cider so that the sugars ferment, turning some of the cider into alcohol.

This alcoholic solution is then further fermented by the addition of bacteria. The result is acetic acid, the main active constituent of unfiltered, unpasteurized vinegar containing the "mother".

Filtered or Unfiltered

Made from apple juice, apple cider vinegar comes in two varieties, filtered or unfiltered. The filtered and pasteurized variety that refines the clear apple cider vinegar removes the sediment and the vinegar mother.

The clear sparkling appearance of filtered, pasteurized apple cider vinegar is more visually appealing to those consumers whose purchasing decisions are driven by aesthetics. Many of these people have been led to believe the misconception that when a product is labeled 'filtered and pasteurized' it is safer and healthier for you.

However with apple cider vinegar, at least, nothing could be further from the truth. As a result of the pasteurizing and filtering process, the healing health-giving properties of raw unpasteurized apple cider are also removed.
The beneficial properties of healthy enzymes and nutrients are filtered out or destroyed by heat during the processing of natural apple cider vinegar.

It is the murky-appearing collection of acetic acid, bacteria and roughage (the mother) that is retained when it is unfiltered and unrefined. It is believed that the live mother in this unfiltered, unpasteurized apple cider vinegar is the reason it has enhanced health-giving properties.

To achieve the maximum health benefits of apple cider vinegar, make sure the label states that the product is both unfiltered and unpasteurized.

Benefits of Apple Cider Vinegar and Honey

The health benefits delivered by natural healers like apple cider vinegar (ACV) and honey are well-known in the holistic health community. In a time where many people would prefer to reach for a pill or chemical to heal what ails them, others are researching natural ways to create the health they crave or maintain what they have.

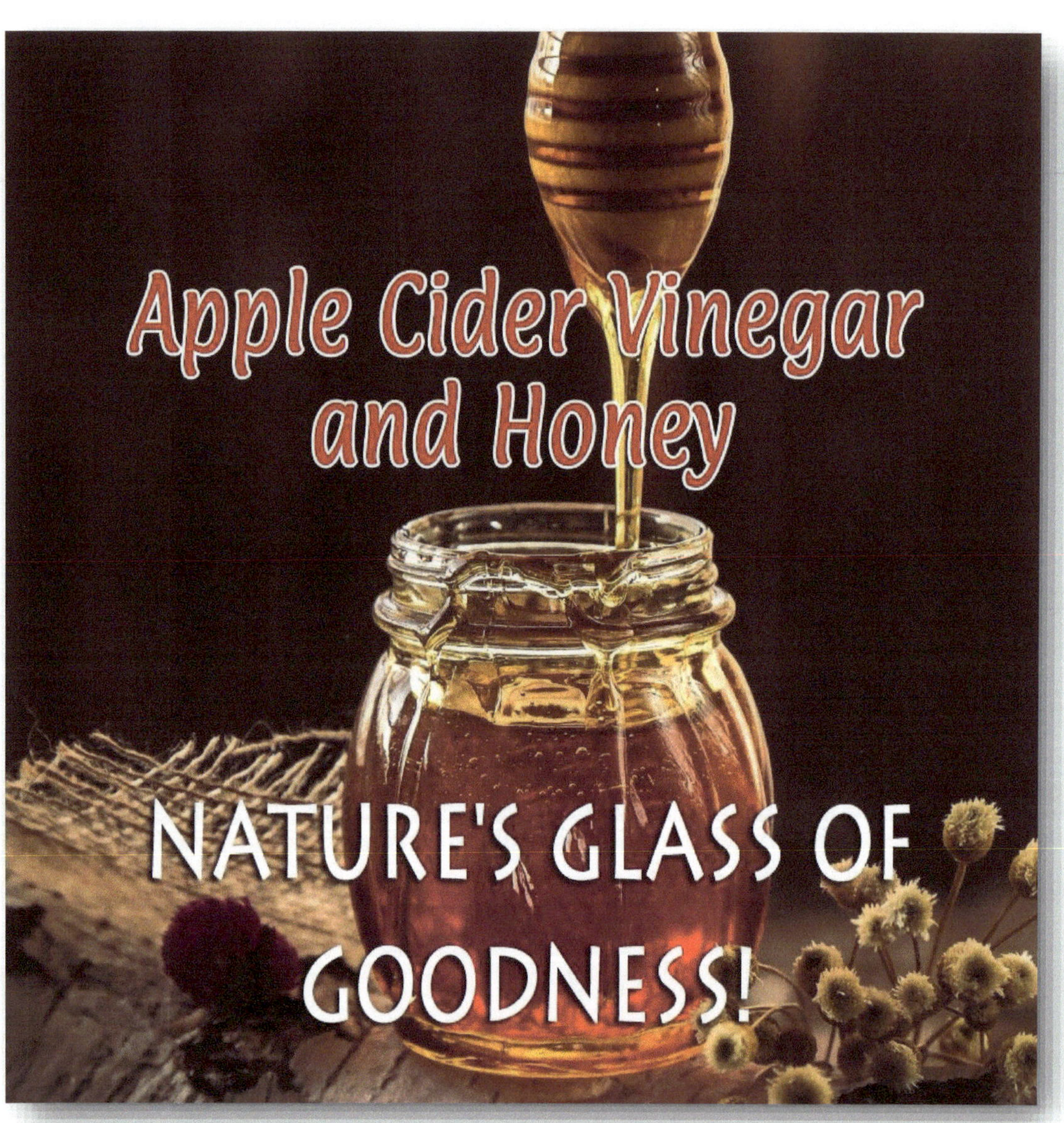

All you have to do is listen to the staggering list of possible side-effects for common prescription and over-the-counter medications to understand the very real need for natural healing methods, which don't offer the possibility of debilitating and dangerous reactions that are often more serious than the illness being treated.

Will an Apple a Day Really Keep the Doctor Away?

There is an old saying that suggests simply eating an apple every day can lead to overall health and wellness. The whole "apple a day keeps the doctor away" premise is based on the multiple positive health attributes associated with eating apples, especially as opposed to processed food.

The soluble dietary fiber in apples can help lower high cholesterol levels, and the polyphenols in apples provide antioxidants which lower high blood pressure and prevent damage to cells in the pancreas.

Eating apples can lower the risk of contracting type 2 diabetes and improve heart health. There are studies which show eating apples regularly can help prevent cancer and regulate digestive health, as well as treat inflammation which is linked to most chronic diseases. When you take the apple superfood and turn it into vinegar, research shows you receive even more health benefits.

A daily apple cider vinegar regimen can enhance your weight loss efforts and improve your skin health. You also receive all of the above-mentioned health benefits. With so many health "gurus" and experts telling you to drink a couple of tablespoons of ACV daily to improve so many health metrics, can you make this natural drink even more powerful by combining it with another well-known natural healer?

Honey – Thousands of Years of Healing

As a natural sweetening alternative to unhealthy refined sugar, raw, unfiltered, and most importantly, unheated honey can't be beat. This natural energy source is packed full of antioxidants which lead to numerous health benefits. Honey promotes the healing of wounds and ulcers, and when you eat locally grown honey, studies show you dramatically reduce your risk of catching colds and flus.

The health properties of honey have been well known for as many as 8,000 years, as evidenced by Stone Age cave drawings which show humans using honey for medicinal and dietary purposes.

Can this ancient natural healer combined with apple cider vinegar, deliver a powerful one-two punch to knock out particular health problems?

The Benefits of an Apple Cider Vinegar and Honey Combo

Each morning when you wake up, make a healthy drink which combines apple cider vinegar, honey and water. This simple morning ritual (which should be practiced before you eat anything, or drink your morning coffee) has powerful anti-inflammatory and pain-fighting properties.

It helps regulate a healthy digestive system, and quickly soothes pain and discomfort in your joints and muscles as well as your throat. The ACV/honey combo helps alkalize the body, bringing your blood back to a naturally healthy pH level.

This means a daily morning dose of honey and ACV helps prevent and manage diseases, fights infections and illness by boosting your immune system, boosts your natural energy levels and has also been linked to healthy weight loss if you are overweight or obese.

This combination of natural health boosters delivers nutrients and vitamins such as pantothenic acid, niacin, folic acid, biotin, pectin, phosphorus and calcium, iron and magnesium, potassium and a long list of B vitamins.

You get significant quantities of acetic and citric acids as well. This combination can also eliminate bad breath, while effectively treating heartburn and acid reflux.

The Magic Dose

How much apple cider vinegar and honey should you be drinking for so many substantial health benefits? The truth is, you don't need much of these proven health promoters to do yourself a world of good. In 8 to 12 ounces of water, add just 1 teaspoon of raw honey and 1 teaspoon of raw, organic ACV.

Drink each morning at least 20 or 30 minutes before you eat anything, and weight loss, heart health, skin improvement and other very real health rewards can be yours.

Apple Cider Vinegar for Lowering Blood Glucose Levels

For hundreds of years vinegar has had a reputation of being a 'must have' pantry product because of its versatility. There are numerous traditional uses such as a food preservative and disinfectant that are well known. Anecdotal claims of the uses and health benefits attributed to apple cider vinegar are wide and varied.

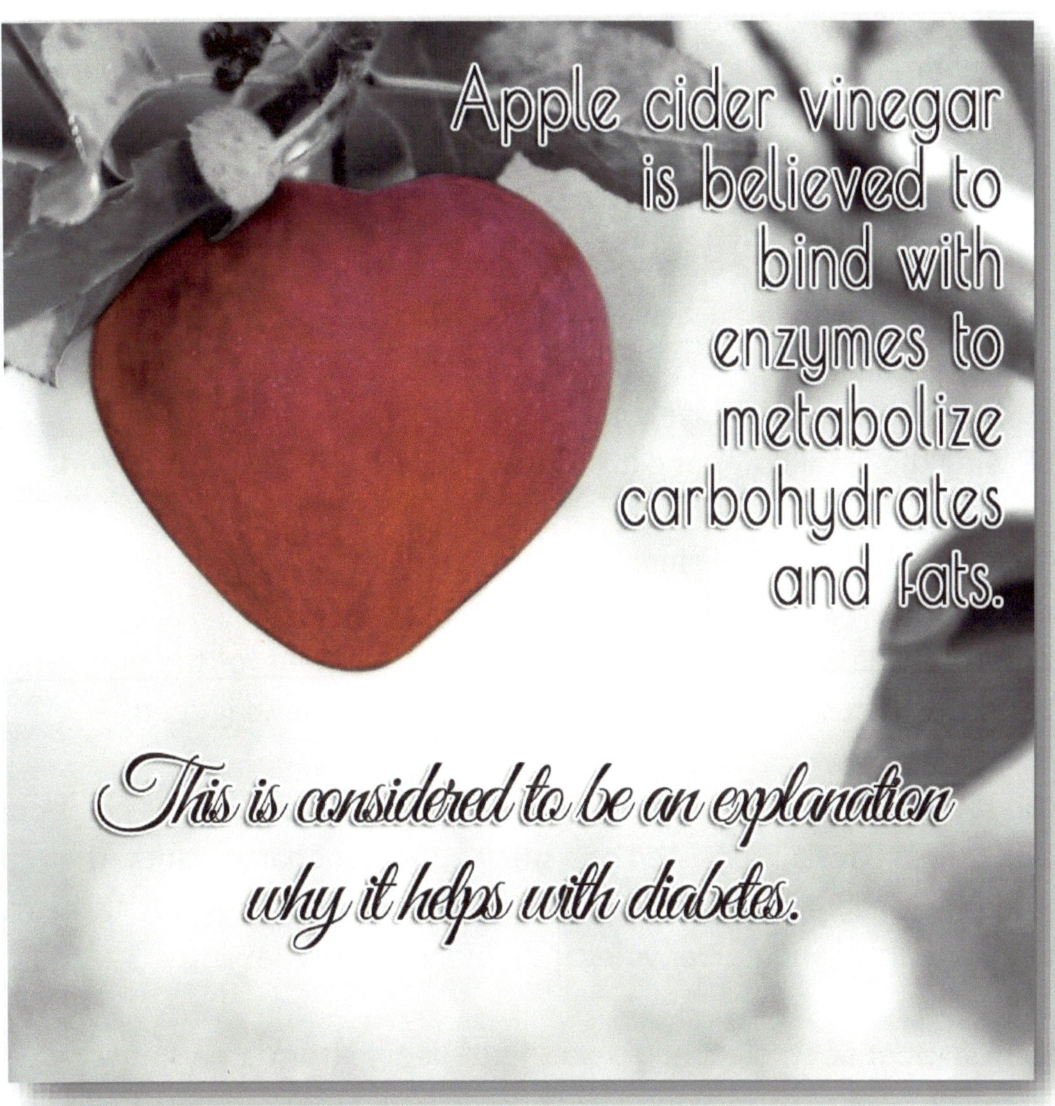

Unfortunately, research and studies into natural health products are not done often enough; therefore many of these claims are not unequivocally supported by science.

Studies Relating to Apple Cider Vinegar and Blood Glucose

One strongly supported claim is that drinking apple cider vinegar before eating and before retiring enables people with diabetes to have better control of their disease. A university study required participants take a drink consisting of apple cider vinegar and water, before each meal.

It was found that those type 2 diabetics with insulin resistance who participated in the trial had 34% lower after-meal glucose levels. Taking the vinegar drink at bedtime has indicated that it promotes insulin production, and therefore lowers the fasting blood glucose levels the following morning.

This study concluded that apple cider vinegar had the same effect on blood glucose levels as pharmaceutical drugs such as acarbose, nateglinide and metformin.

These drugs control blood sugar levels in sufferers of type 2 diabetes. They work in the intestine, slowing the breakdown and absorption of carbohydrates from food.

Apple cider vinegar is believed to bind with enzymes to metabolize carbs and fats. This is considered to be an explanation why it helps with diabetes.
If the potential of apple cider vinegar being a natural treatment for the prevention or control of type 2 diabetes is realized, it would be very good news indeed.

Although the studies conducted to date have been positive, researchers point out that the study and others have all consisted of a small number of participants. They conclude that unless a large randomized trial is conducted it will be difficult to verify the true potential and benefits of apple cider vinegar on blood glucose levels.

However lack of scientific studies should not deter people from experimenting with apple cider vinegar. Plenty of anecdotal evidence praising the countless health benefits of this versatile product is widely available. It is claimed by many to be the most effective panacea as a home remedy available.

Is Apple Cider Vinegar Safe?

Apple cider vinegar is in itself considered safe and there is no recommended dosage. Reputable sources suggest up to a tablespoon three or four times a day, and that it should be taken diluted with water.

However, because of the possible interaction with medication you may already be taking, it is recommended that you consult your health professional before trying anything new.

Apple cider vinegar is reputed to decrease blood glucose levels. Medication for people with diabetes is designed to lower blood sugar levels. Combining both insulin and apple cider vinegar could cause blood glucose levels to drop too low, resulting in temporary hypoglycemia. Closely monitored blood glucose levels will reveal if insulin medication needs to be adjusted.

Insulin sometimes has the effect of decreasing the amount of potassium in the body. Taking large doses of apple cider vinegar also has the potential to reduce potassium levels. Therefore insulin dependent people should avoid large doses of apple cider vinegar in combination with their insulin medication.

What Apple Cider Vinegar Should You Use?

If your doctor permits, choose the organic, unfiltered, unpasteurized and raw product. It may be murky and often contains a substance called the mother, which are brown-like strands that resemble cobwebs. This natural vinegar contains enzymes and healthy bacteria and is considered to contain the most health benefits.

Apple Cider Vinegar for Skin Conditions

It is well known that skin health comes from within. The buildup of toxins in the body prevents the liver and other organs from working efficiently. A congested liver can result in a hormone imbalance, constipation and digestive problems.

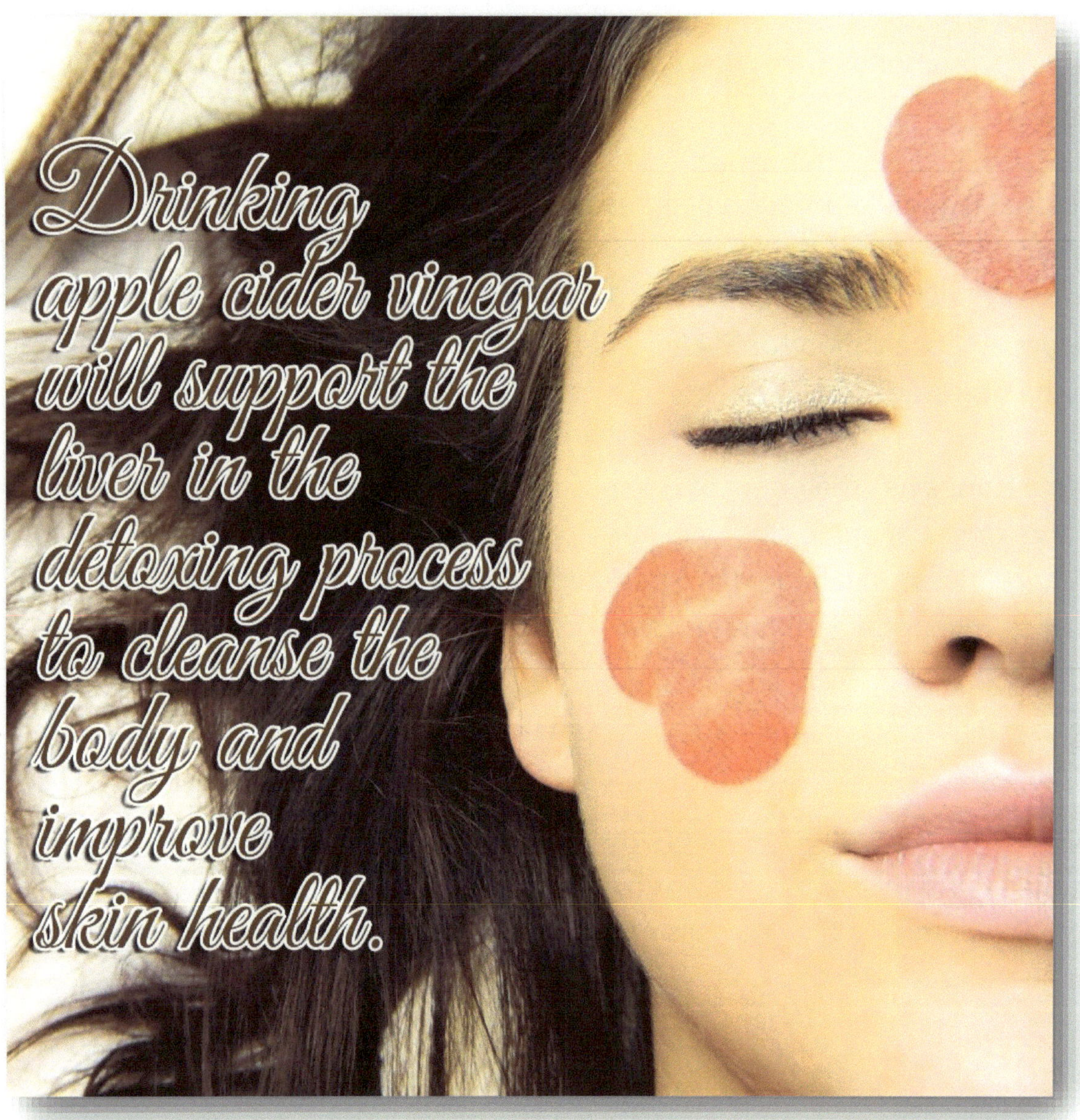

When toxins build up because the normal elimination organs cannot handle the load, the body will try to excrete them via the skin. Itching, rashes and other skin disorders are the body's reaction to accumulated excess toxins.

The Benefits of Detoxification

Drinking apple cider vinegar will support the liver in the detoxing process to cleanse the body. This will improve circulation, purify the blood and relieve constipation by more efficiently removing waste from the body.

Until the liver is cleansed and the balance restored, the effectiveness of topical applications to skin disorders will be minimal. This is of particular importance to sufferers of hormonal acne and candida.

Apple cider vinegar can be taken both orally and also used as a topical medication to treat many skin conditions. However the cider vinegar must be unpasteurized, unfiltered, and ideally with the mother still intact.

Unlike the pasteurized variety this raw vinegar still contains all the rich natural goodness. It is full of healthy bacteria, protein, acetic acid and amazing enzymes. One of the health benefits of drinking apple cider vinegar is the ability it has to detoxify the body.

There is no specific dose for taking apple cider vinegar but common doses range from 1-2 teaspoons to 1-2 tablespoons in a glass of water or fruit juice, preferably taken before meals. It can also be used in cooking or salad dressings.

Using as a dressing, without the application of heat, is a healthy and tasty way to consume apple cider vinegar, without making it seem like a 'medicine'.

There are many different skin disorders, and many can be helped with applying apple cider vinegar. These include acne, pimples, rashes, hives and warts.

Facial Skin Toner and Topical Medication

Here is a recipe for an economical and very effective skin toner that not only replaces your expensive store bought facial toner but is also a topical medication for many skin ailments. Combine one-part raw apple cider vinegar with two parts of distilled or filtered water, that's it. Apply to skin!

Fermented raw apple cider vinegar has lots of pectin, calcium and is fortified with even more beneficial enzymes and acids. So, applying this mixture after cleansing your face not only tones the skin but will improve skin conditions such pimples, acne, and acne scars. It has also been found to lighten sun and age spots.

Topical Application for Other Skin Aliments

Warts

Warts are a viral growth on the skin that can be treated with apple cider vinegar. Apply the vinegar to the warts each night and cover them with a band-aid. Leave uncovered during the day. Repeat this every day and results will be seen in about a week or a little longer.

Sunburn

A cupful of apple cider vinegar added to your bath will neutralize the burn and soothe the sunburn.

Rashes and Itches

Yeast infections, hives, skin rashes and itchy skin can all be relieved by the addition of apple cider vinegar in the bath.

Containing antiseptic and antibacterial properties, apple cider vinegar is very beneficial as a topical medication when dealing with skin infections and conditions like eczema, dermatitis, and psoriasis.

As emphasized above all skin disorders have their origin from within. Apple cider vinegar taken orally improves liver function, keeps the gut healthy and benefits overall health, while topical applications soothe and help to heal the skin itself.

Apple Cider Vinegar for Colds

The common cold is a condition that affects the upper respiratory tract. Symptoms may include a sore throat, sneezing, fever, runny nose and headache, and 'getting a cold' is considered a common occurrence, especially during a cold and/or rainy season.

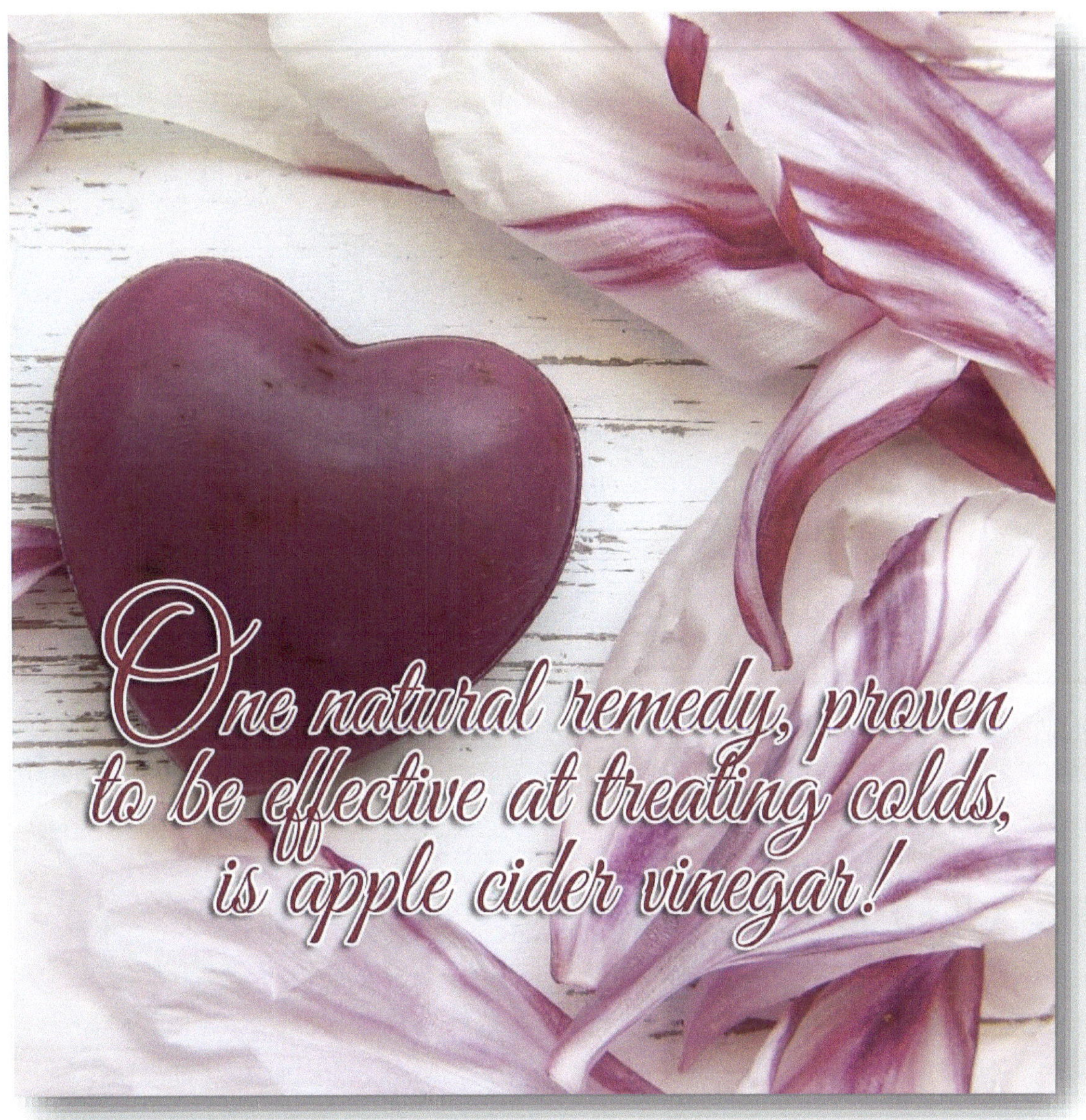

However, you don't have to reach for prescription medications. One natural remedy, proven to be effective at treating colds, is apple cider vinegar.

Apple Cider Vinegar Has Antimicrobial Properties

The active compounds present in apple juice, apple cider and apple cider vinegar have been shown to have antiviral properties. They may not be able to completely destroy all cold viruses, but they can significantly reduce the severity of the attack, and thereby reduce subsequent symptoms and infections.

Although a virus is what causes the initial infection, the symptoms from the infection will usually last for approximately two days only. However, as you would no doubt know, most colds last for several days or more.

This is because the cells in the airways, damaged by the virus infection, become highly susceptible to a secondary infection. This secondary infection is now caused by the bacteria present.

The pre-existing bacteria in the airway cells normally don't cause any problems. However, once these cells are killed by a virus and the tissues become inflamed, there is an increase in the numbers of disease-causing pathogens.

The acetic acid content of apple cider vinegar is capable of passing into the cell membranes of the micro-organisms. This leads to bacterial cell death. In simple terms, the antimicrobial properties found in apple cider vinegar is what makes it helpful in fighting against the common cold. It helps provide relief from cold symptoms by killing the bacteria that cause them.

ACV Has Alkalizing Properties

Cold viruses have the potential to put the body into a very acidic state, which makes the body more conducive to the continued reproduction of the virus, as well as the secondary bacterial infections. As a result, the immune system has a hard time fighting against the 'infection invasion'.

Apple cider vinegar is a powerful alkalizing substance that can defeat the cold symptom-causing micro-organisms, providing relief from the symptoms. The acidic nature of apple cider vinegar inhibits bacterial growth, and this prevents the infection from spreading and becoming worse.

Other Benefits of Apple Cider Vinegar If You Have a Cold

ACV contains several nutrients and enzymes that aid in strengthening the immune system. This of course helps a person to be better able to fight against virus infections, including the common cold.

Apple cider vinegar has also been found effective in breaking up thick mucus, caused by colds, as well as helping relieve sinusitis and cough.

How to Use ACV for Treating Colds Fast

There are plenty of ways that apple cider vinegar can be used when treating colds. Here are a few ways you can use ACV to provide rapid and effective relief.

ACV with Lemon and Honey

Mix 2 tablespoons of ACV in a glass of warm water. Add in lemon and honey and drink this solution as often as needed.

Add ACV to Steam (Or In Your Vaporizer)

Another way to treat colds using ACV is to add a few drops into a vaporizer. This can greatly relieve the symptoms of colds, flu and other infections.

You may also use ACV in a bowl of steaming water. Just add a few teaspoons of ACV into a bowl of boiling water before inhaling the steam.

ACV with Garlic

Put one cup of ACV, eight cloves of garlic and a cup of honey into a blender. Pour the mixture into a glass and drink as required. If you want to drink it cold, refrigerate first before drinking.

ACV Brew

Drinking an apple cider vinegar brew is one great way to get rid of common cold symptoms. To make an ACV brew, mix ¼ cup of ACV in a glass of hot water. Add one tablespoon of honey and one teaspoon of cayenne pepper. Mix well. Then add a few drops of lemon before drinking.

Apple cider vinegar is a great remedy to keep on hand to boost your immune system and to keep colds away!

Apple Cider Vinegar for Gout

Gout is a form of arthritis, known as 'Gouty Arthritis'. It occurs due to the buildup of uric acid in the joints. Symptoms of this condition include redness, swelling, tenderness and severe episodes of pain. This condition usually affects the big toe.

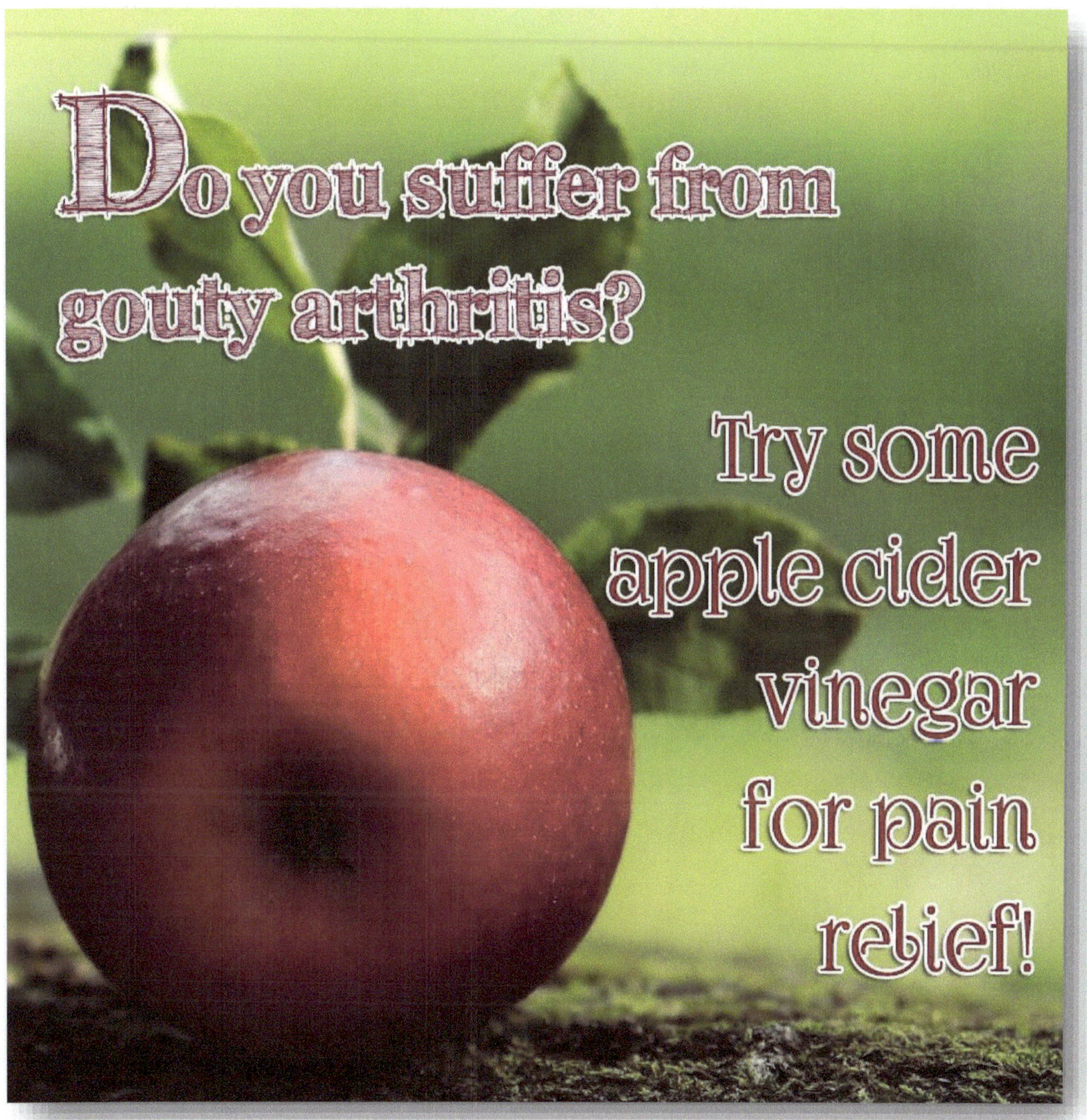

Eliminating alcohol and foods that can increase uric acid in the body are two important steps in reducing gout symptoms. However, there is also one effective natural remedy that can be used by gout sufferers. This remedy is apple cider vinegar. ACV can bring gout sufferers relief from gout pain.

Apple Cider Vinegar Promotes Alkalinity

Acetic acid is the main substance found in ACV that makes it beneficial for those who have gout pain. Although it is considered as acidic, acetic acid becomes alkaline once inside the body.

In turn, a pH-balanced environment is formed inside the body. Maintaining an alkaline environment in the body is crucial to the process of getting rid of gout symptoms. Once the alkaline levels are maintained, gout symptoms will less likely recur.

According to Dr. Theodore Baroody, the author of *"Alkalize or Die"*, during the initial phase of using ACV to treat gout, the symptoms may increase. This occurs as a reaction to the uric acid.

It actually causes inflammation while the acid crystals are being dissolved. However, within weeks these reactions will eventually subside.

Here are some other reasons why ACV is beneficial for people who have gout:

- Its malic acid content works to neutralize then dissolve uric acid.
- It contains potassium that aids in waste elimination.
- Its amino acids have been found to result in lowered levels of toxicity.

Gout sufferers may need to take larger amounts of ACV in order to experience relief from their symptoms. It may be necessary to take two tablespoons of ACV up to three times a day.

Some people experience relief from their symptoms of gout within a couple of hours of taking ACV. Others claim to have experienced relief only after a few days of taking ACV.

If you take apple cider vinegar and experience an upset stomach then avoid taking it again or take in a very small amount to see if you are still affected.

Taking a 'Shot' of Apple Cider Vinegar

Gout can bring about debilitating pain, and to ease the pain rapidly many take a 'shot glass' of ACV and then follow it up immediately with a glass of water.

Drinking plenty of water after taking ACV is important, as gout symptoms can also worsen with dehydration. Drinking plenty water also helps the body get rid of toxins and uric acid crystals.

Other Ways of Using ACV for Gout

If you find it hard to take a shot glass of undiluted ACV, you may add two teaspoons to other juices. One extra special juice to add your ACV to is cherry juice. Cherry juice has been shown to help alleviate gout symptoms for some people. So if you add ACV to cherry juice, you may just have a 'double dose' of relief.

In conjunction to taking apple cider vinegar orally, ACV can also be applied topically. Here are a few examples on how ACV can be used topically for the gout relief.

- To prevent gout attacks in the middle of the night, try an ACV wrap. Use an old clean cloth and soak it in apple cider vinegar. Then, wrap the cloth on the affected area. Cover the cloth with a plastic wrap and a bandage to prevent it from slipping off while you sleep.

- Pour ACV into a spray bottle and then spray it to the affected area. You may also choose to place the spray bottle in the refrigerator. The coolness of the ACV is an added relief for gout pain. You can do this every hour until the pain subsides.

- Pour ACV into ice cube trays and place in the freezer. Apply the cubes to the affected area.

Don't forget, when you buy apple cider vinegar to use orally, choose the one that is unfiltered and unpasteurized.

Apple Cider Vinegar for Weight Loss

If you are looking to lose weight, there is one simple habit that may be worth adding to your weight loss regimen. This is the inclusion of apple cider vinegar in your diet.

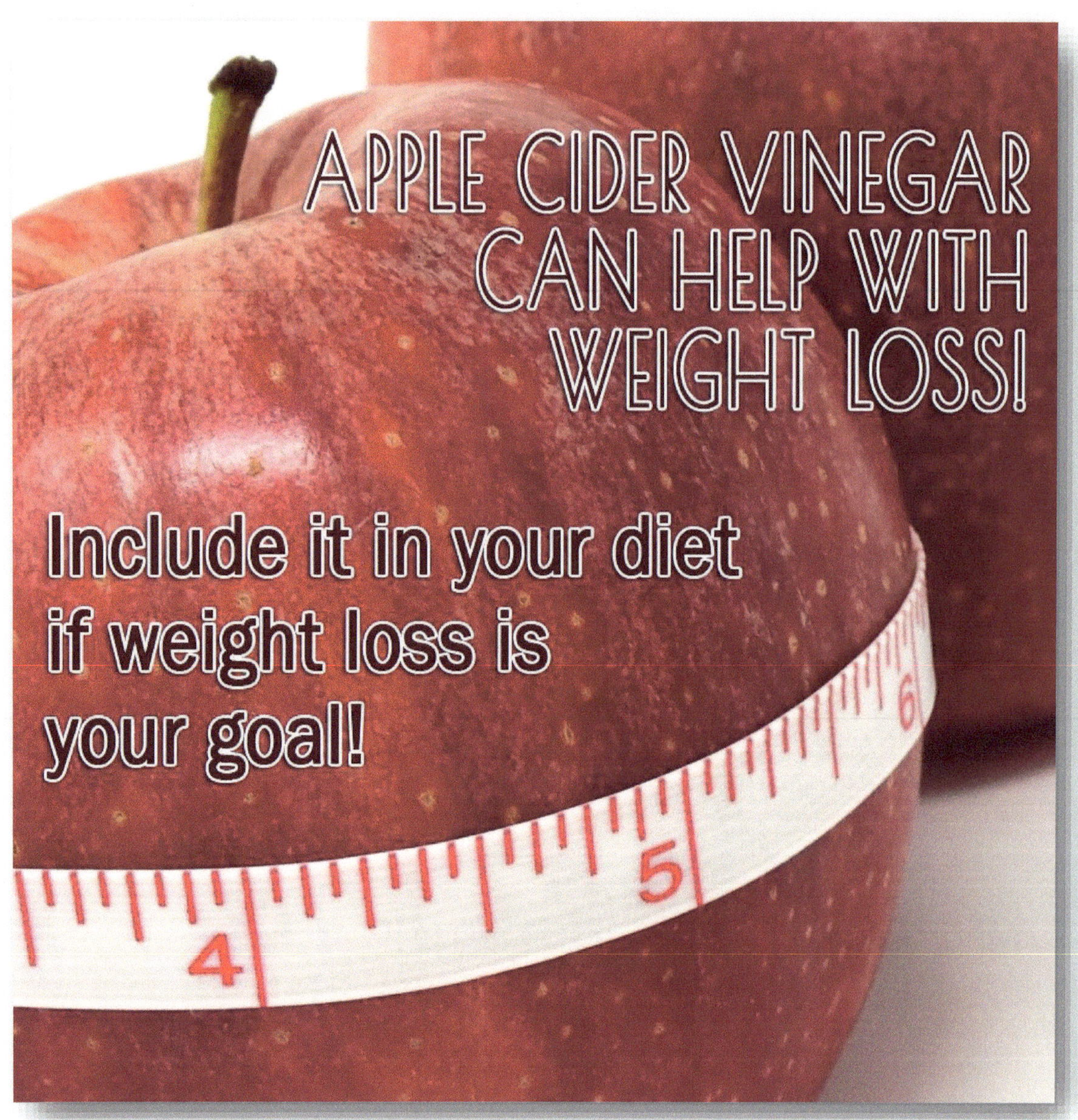

Whether you dilute it in a glass of water or pour it on your salad, apple cider vinegar is definitely worth a try!

Here are the reasons why apple cider vinegar helps you lose weight.

ACV Promotes Satiety, Reduces Caloric Consumption

The acetic acid content of apple cider vinegar is capable of blocking disaccharides. By taking ACV before eating, disaccharides from carbohydrates are prevented from being easily absorbed into the bloodstream. This habit reduces the onset of sugar spikes, which are usually experienced after eating a meal loaded with sugar or carbohydrates.

A small study which only had 11 participants showed that those who consumed apple cider vinegar with their high-carb meal were found to have lowered their blood sugar response up to 55%. This means when acetic acid is consumed the body's insulin response to carbohydrates, such as bread and biscuits, slows down.

A study showed that those who ate bread and included ACV with their meal, experienced better satiety levels than those who only ate the bread. Researchers found that the caloric consumption of study participants were between 200 to 275 fewer calories than those who did not take ACV.

This affect is good news for those who want to lose weight.

Achieving satiety is important for eliminating the tendency to overeat, snack between meals and crave too many sugar-laden foods. Along with satiety, ACV also provides appetite-suppressant properties that contribute to the reduction of overall caloric consumption.

The Importance of Hormones in Weight Loss

Apple cider vinegar has been shown to help the body more efficiently digest protein. Efficient protein digestion is necessary for effective weight management and overall health. It is also essential for optimum hormone production.

Protein is a crucial macronutrient that the body needs for the formation of growth hormones. Proteins are required while growth hormone formation takes place. This process continues to occur even when the person is at rest. In other words, the body needs to keep on burning energy to fuel this body process.

If you take apple cider vinegar before a meal, the digestion of proteins and hormone synthesis will more efficiently take place.

Hormones serve as chemical messengers to promote the proper functioning of almost all processes that take place in the body. If our hormones get out of balance – there is a breakdown in 'internal body communication'.

Proper communication between hormones is crucial towards helping a person lose weight. Without proper communication these hormones may have difficulty determining whether the body needs to lose weight or gain weight, or whether it should be storing or burning more fats.

ACV Helps Stimulate Digestion

If the digestive system is stimulated, it is less likely to become sluggish. It is important for food to stay in the digestive tract only long enough for proper nutrient absorption, however, excess or unwanted fats and toxins that stay too long in the digestive tract will be absorbed by the body.

Apple cider vinegar can help prevent this occurrence by stimulating the digestion process. This lessens the amount of time that excess fats remain in the digestive tract.

ACV Speeds Up Metabolism

One reason why ACV is used for weight loss is that it helps utilize body fat. Research reveals that ACV can speed up metabolism, burn fat and prevent fat storage in the body. This is attributed to the acid content of ACV which has the ability to increase fat burning enzymes. These are also the type of enzymes that help decrease sugar and fat storage.

A study of obese participants showed the effectiveness of ACV in promoting weight loss. These study participants were grouped into three. The first group were given one tablespoon of vinegar. The second group had two tablespoons of vinegar. The third group were given a placebo. The results showed that those who consumed vinegar were found to lose more weight compared to the placebo group after a twelve-week period.

ACV Boosts Tryptophan Production

When proteins are released during the process of digestion, the production of tryptophan also improves. Tryptophan is an amino acid that is important for weight loss. It is essential in making a person feel more satisfied. Tryptophan also acts as a precursor for serotonin production. Serotonin is also referred to as the "feel-good" hormone. As serotonin promotes feelings of satisfaction, overeating and cravings will be better kept at bay, and comfort eating reduced.

ACV Aids in Natural Detoxification

Apple cider vinegar is beneficial for promoting regular bowel movements. Therefore, it helps to improve the body's ability to get rid of toxins. Regular bowel movements are important to prevent waste from building up in the digestive tract. The toxins are then less likely to recirculate into the bloodstream and be reabsorbed which may result in weight gain.

Although ACV may aid in a person's weight loss efforts, it doesn't replace healthy eating habits or regular exercise. It is a healthy addition to your diet. Remember to consume apple cider vinegar in moderation.

Apple Cider Vinegar Side Effects

Apple cider vinegar is made from fermented crushed apples and is considered by many as being a safe, natural product. It contains pectin, biotin, pantothenic acid, vitamins and minerals. It is also known for its acetic acid which has earned a reputation for relieving the symptoms of several illnesses.

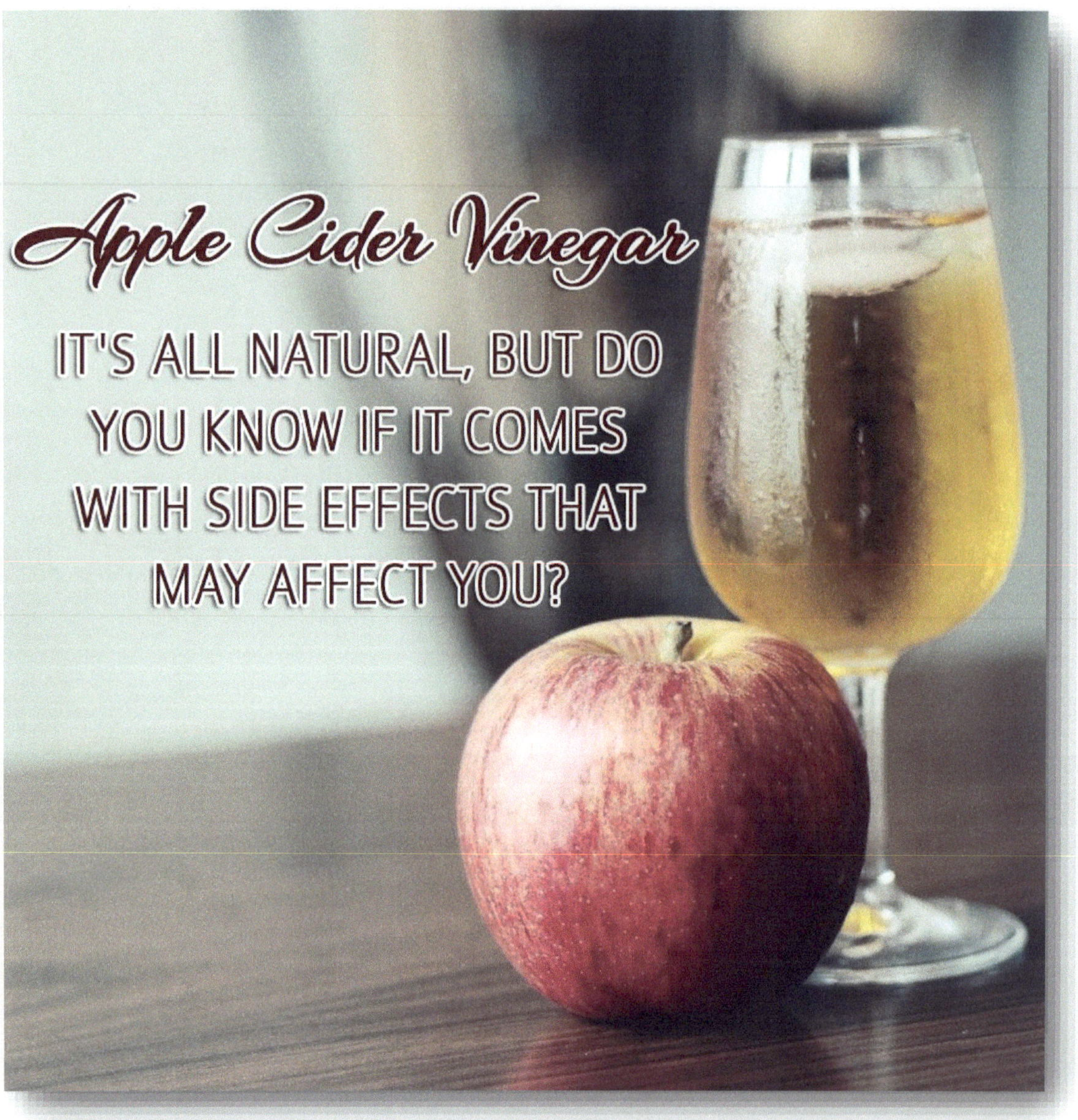

However, regular intake of apple cider vinegar can also bring about some adverse side affects you should be aware of.

Throat Irritation

Throat irritation is the most common side effect of regular and prolonged consumption of apple cider vinegar. This is because of its acetic acid content. To prevent throat irritation, it is best to dilute ACV into a glass of water to avoid burning the esophageal wall.

Enamel Erosion

The acid content of ACV may cause tooth enamel to erode. This increases the risk of tooth decay. Although the saliva in the mouth serves to buffer the acidity of the vinegar, evidence from studies show that taking large amounts of vinegar can lead to dental erosion.

Blood Sugar Problems

ACV is found to have an anti-glycemic effect, which means it can help lower blood sugar levels. This may seem beneficial for many, or even most people, however, for some people this anti-glycemic effect can be a problem. Taking in ACV may cause blood glucose levels to drop too low, which may trigger the onset of diabetic hypoglycemia.

If you have a pre-existing history of hypoglycemia (low blood sugar), consult your physician first before taking ACV.

Digestive Problems and Type 1 Diabetes

Apple cider vinegar has been shown to help prevent the onset of blood sugar spikes improve insulin sensitivity. It can also reduce the rate at which the food moves from the stomach into the lower digestive tract, which makes a person feel fuller, longer.

A study showed that taking 2 tablespoons of apple cider vinegar mixed in a glass of water, can reduce the emptying rate of the stomach. This can be beneficial for those who experience blood sugar spikes, or for those trying to lose weight.

However, the effect may worsen the symptoms of gastroparesis, which usually affects individuals with type 1 diabetes. Gastroparesis is a condition that occurs when the stomach is not working at an optimum level.

This means the stomach is not emptied properly at a normal rate and the food stays in the stomach longer than is desirable. Symptoms of gastroparesis include nausea, bloating and heartburn.

Individuals with type 1 diabetes should seek medical advice before taking apple cider vinegar.

Drug Interactions

Extra precautions must be taken by those who are taking prescription medications for their existing medical conditions. Below are just a few examples of medications that may cause adverse reactions when taken along with apple cider vinegar.

- *Digoxin (Lanoxin)*

This drug lowers the potassium levels in the body. Therefore, if this is taken along with apple cider vinegar it may increase the risk of having very low levels of potassium.

- *Diabetes Medications*

Taking ACV while maintaining insulin-stimulating drugs can be dangerous as it can cause very low blood sugar levels. Symptoms of low blood sugar include heart palpitations, dizziness, nervousness and trembling. If left untreated, it can lead to seizure and loss of consciousness.

- *Diuretic Drugs*

Diuretic drugs trigger the body to excrete more potassium. Therefore, if a person also takes apple cider vinegar, their potassium may drop to dangerously low levels.

Bottom Line

For most people, apple cider vinegar is a very beneficial tonic. It helps keep infection away and helps with maintaining healthy weight.

Those with type 1 diabetes or who are taking certain medications should take advice and care before using ACV.

Others have reported problems when used to excess over long periods, or when used undiluted. So, a couple of teaspoons mixed with water, a few times a day should not cause problems for most.

Can Drinking Apple Cider Vinegar Daily Be Good for You?

Drinking apple cider vinegar with water is a healthy habit that most people can incorporate into your daily routine.

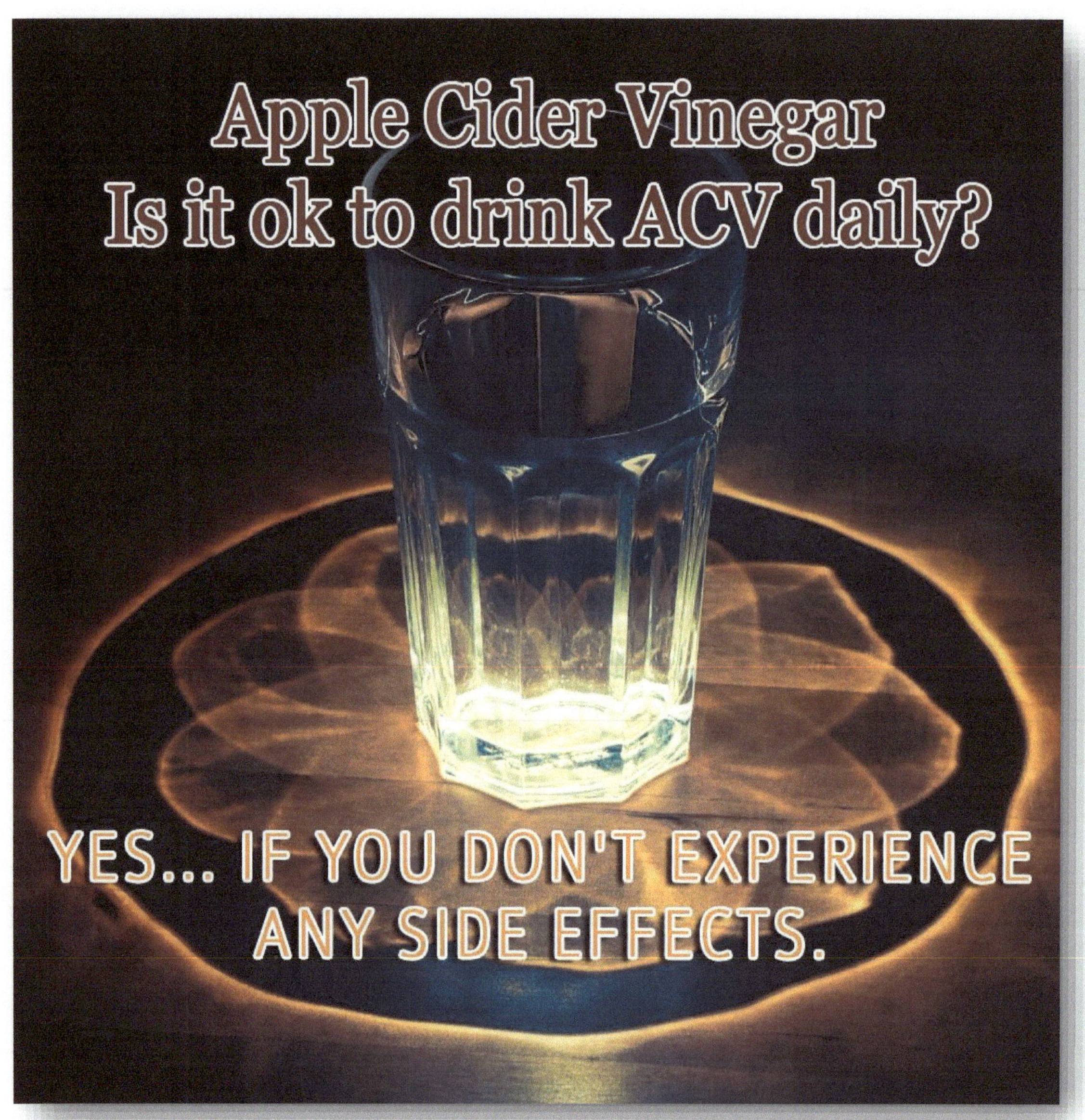

However, you should not take more than two tablespoons of apple cider vinegar every day, and always remember to dilute it with water. Diluting it will make it less acidic for your esophagus.

Drinking diluted ACV on a daily basis can provide several health benefits.

Helps manage type 2 diabetes

Vinegar has been found by experts to help improve insulin sensitivity. Insulin sensitivity is crucial towards achieving lower blood sugar. Studies reveal that vinegar leads to a significant buffering of blood sugar levels, even after indulging in a heavy carbohydrate meal.

Studies have also shown that adding apple cider vinegar to salad dressings can also help lower blood sugar levels.

Experts confirm that taking 2 tablespoons of ACV can help improve fasting blood sugar by up to 4%, however, if you have been diagnosed with diabetes (especially type 1), it is wise to check with your physician first before taking ACV.

Feel more satiated

In one study, participants were given white bread and vinegar, however, not all participants consumed the same level of vinegar. Some participants were given vinegar with low levels of acetic acid. Others were given vinegar with higher levels of acetic acid. The results showed that those who were given higher levels of acetic acid were found to feel fuller than the other participants.

Your skin will improve

Apple cider vinegar is also known to improve skin health as it reduces scarring and helps treat acne. Bacteria is usually the culprit for acne and other skin problems. The benefit found in the apple cider vinegar is that it contains antibacterial properties, effective in fighting against bacterial skin infections.

Lowers your risk of heart disease

Since ACV helps lower blood pressure, it can also help reduce the risk of heart disease. ACV also aids in increasing good cholesterol levels and helpful in regulating triglyceride levels. These findings have been confirmed in several studies.

It aids in regular bowel movement

ACV is also known to act as a natural laxative. Many people who drink it on a regular basis claim to have improved bowel movements. This effect can be attributed to its water-soluble content of pectin.

Drinking a glass of water mixed with 2 teaspoons of ACV have been found effective in relieving the symptoms of irritable bowel syndrome or IBS. This condition has been linked to having low levels of stomach acid. This is when ACV is helpful for it contains acetic acid which has alkalizing effect once in the digestive system.

You may experience less heartburn.

Stomach acid that is produced for digestion should remain in the stomach. The muscles at the entrance of the stomach must close and open at the right time. However, this doesn't happen when heartburn or acid reflux is experienced.

Unfortunately, some people's stomach muscles do not perform the way they should, and this is when they experience acid reflux or heartburn. Taking apple cider vinegar can help reduce heartburn. It is because ACV contains acetic acid that when ingested becomes capable of alkalizing the stomach environment.

This keeps the symptoms of acid reflux at bay.

Although the acid content of ACV provides health benefits, extra precautions must still be taken. Some people can experience side effects, so always check with your health care professional if you have any concerns.

Conclusion

Apple cider vinegar has been shown repeatedly to be effective in managing many health problems, but still has its doubters and detractors.

Perhaps they should do a little research into the use of ACV and animal health. Apple cider vinegar is greatly used by many commercial and recreational animal owners.

These are people who won't continue spending money on products that don't work, they keep using it because it does. With animals, ACV has been tested and proven without the constraints applied to human pharmacology.

Applied topically or taken internally (depending on the ailment) it provides an inexpensive remedy.

Very little care is needed regarding dosage, as it has a wide margin of safety. It is a powerful product, though, and for most uses is best diluted with water.

Beet- Pickled Deviled Eggs

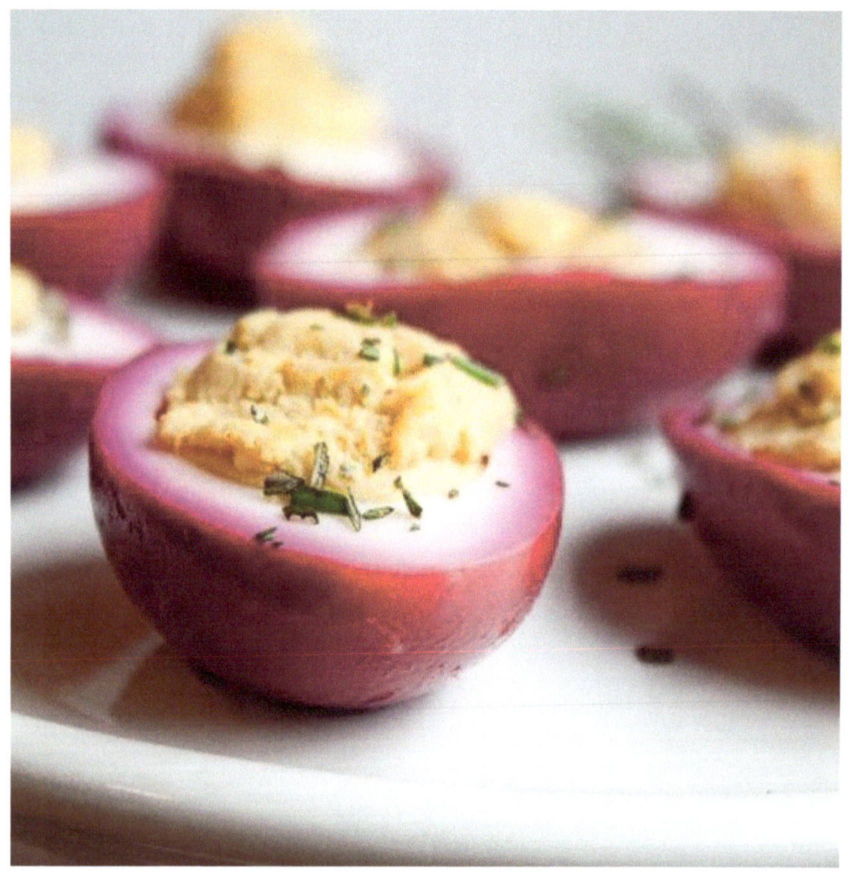

You'll add the apple cider vinegar to the beet brine to make these brilliantly colored deviled eggs.

Makes 12

Ingredients:

- 6 large eggs
- 1 16-ounce can or jar pickled beets
- 1 cup apple cider vinegar
- 1/3 cup brown sugar
- 1 tablespoon peppercorns
- 1 teaspoon salt
- 1 teaspoon Dijon mustard
- 1 tablespoon mayonnaise
- 1/2 teaspoon curry powder
- 1 tablespoon vinegar
- 2 tablespoons olive oil
- Salt and pepper to taste
- Fresh rosemary for garnish

Instructions:

1. Hard boil your eggs. Remove the shells and set the eggs aside.
2. Prepare the brine. Pour a can of pickled beets in a large bowl or mason jar. Add apple cider vinegar, sugar, peppercorns, and salt. Stir.
3. Put the peeled eggs into the brine carefully.
4. Cover and refrigerate for at least 12 hours, or up to 3 days. The longer you leave them in the brine, the more sour and pink they'll end up.
5. After the brining time, cut each egg in half. Scoop out the yolks and place them in a medium-sized bowl, along with mayonnaise, mustard, curry, vinegar, and olive oil.
6. Mash and mix until smooth.
7. If the mixture is too stiff, add a little water.
8. Add salt and pepper to taste.
9. Pipe the yolk mixture back into the pink eggs using a pastry bag.
10. Sprinkle with chopped rosemary.

Apple Cabbage Salad with Cider Vinaigrette

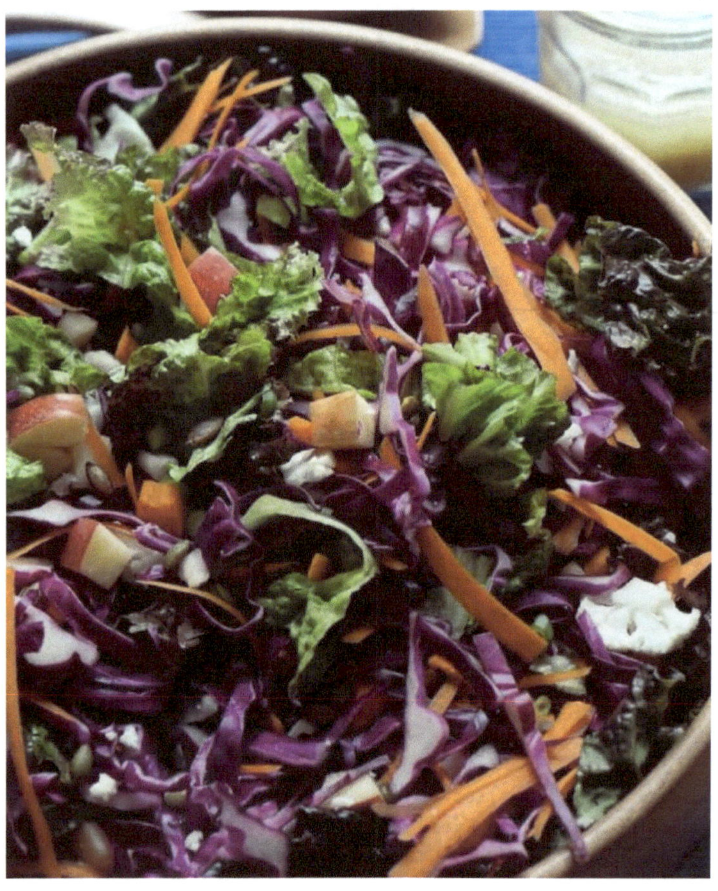

The cider vinegar in the dressing helps cut through the rich flavors of the meat.

Serves 4 to 6

Ingredients:

- 5 cups thinly sliced red cabbage (about 1/4 of one medium head)
- 4 ounces lettuce (about half of a small head), torn or sliced into strips
- 2 medium apples (crunchy, crisp varieties like Honeycrip, Gala, or SweeTango), diced small
- 2 medium carrots, peeled into ribbons
- 2 cups finely chopped cauliflower (pull off about 3 of the cumulus cloud shaped bunches from the head, cut away the thick stem, and then chop the florets into tinier bits)
- 1/2 cup thinly sliced scallions, green and white parts (about 3 or 4 scallions)
- 3 tablespoons canola, vegetable, safflower, or a mild nut oil like almond or walnut
- 1 1/2 tablespoons mayonnaise
- 1 1/2 teaspoons brown sugar (light or dark)
- 1/4 teaspoon Dijon mustard
- 3 tablespoons apple cider vinegar
- Pinch of fine sea salt
- 5 grinds fresh black pepper
- 1/2 cup pepitas, toasted

Instructions:

1. Combine the cabbage, lettuce, apples, carrots, cauliflower, and scallions in a large serving bowl. Toss several times so that the carrot ribbons tangle with the cabbage shreds and lettuce leaves, and the cubes of apples and bits of cauliflower settle throughout rather than at the bottom of the bowl.
2. Briskly whisk together the mayonnaise and oil until smooth. Add the mustard and sugar, then whisk again. Then, whip in the vinegar, salt, and pepper until the whole of it emulsifies into one dressing.
3. Pour the vinaigrette over the salad, scatter the pepitas, and toss again to combine everything.
4. Serve immediately.

Notes:

If you plan on having leftovers, hold off on the vinaigrette and pepitas, adding those per serving to prevent the salad from becoming soggy and the pepitas from losing their crispy crunch (You can just reserve a portion of the salad for saving, too, and dress the rest for serving immediately).

Refrigerate the undressed salad in an airtight container for up to 4 days and store the pepitas in a zip-top bag or container outside of the fridge.

Sardine Snacking Toasts

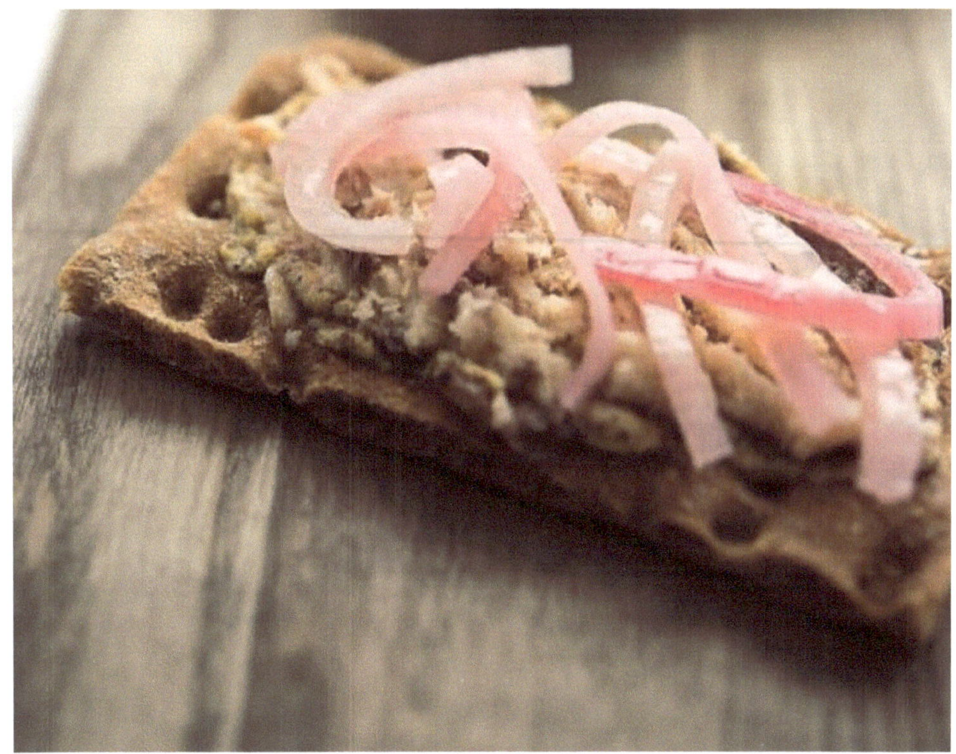

The apple cider vinegar comes into play in this recipe in the form of pickled red onions, which sit atop the sardine spread.

Makes 4 toasts

Ingredients:

For the pickled onions:

- 1 small red onion (about 5 ounces)
- 1/2 cup apple cider vinegar
- 1/2 cup water
- 1/2 teaspoon granulated sugar
- 1/2 teaspoon fine salt

For the toasts:

- 4 Wasa crispbreads
- 4 teaspoons Dijon mustard
- 1 (3.5 ounce) can sardines

Instructions:

For the pickled onions:

1. Peel and cut the onion lengthwise. Thinly slice the halves and set aside.
2. Bring the vinegar, water, sugar, and salt to a boil in a medium saucepan over medium-high heat, stirring to dissolve the salt and sugar.
3. Remove from the heat, add the onion, and stir to combine. Make sure all the onions are submerged. Let it sit for 15 minutes before using and store in an airtight container. Put inside the refrigerator. This can last for up to 1 month.

For the toasts:

1. Spread a teaspoon of mustard on each crisp bread.
2. Divide the sardines among the crisp breads and gently smash into an even layer with the back of a fork.
3. Place a thin layer of pickled red onions over the sardines
4. Serve immediately.

Collard Green Slaw

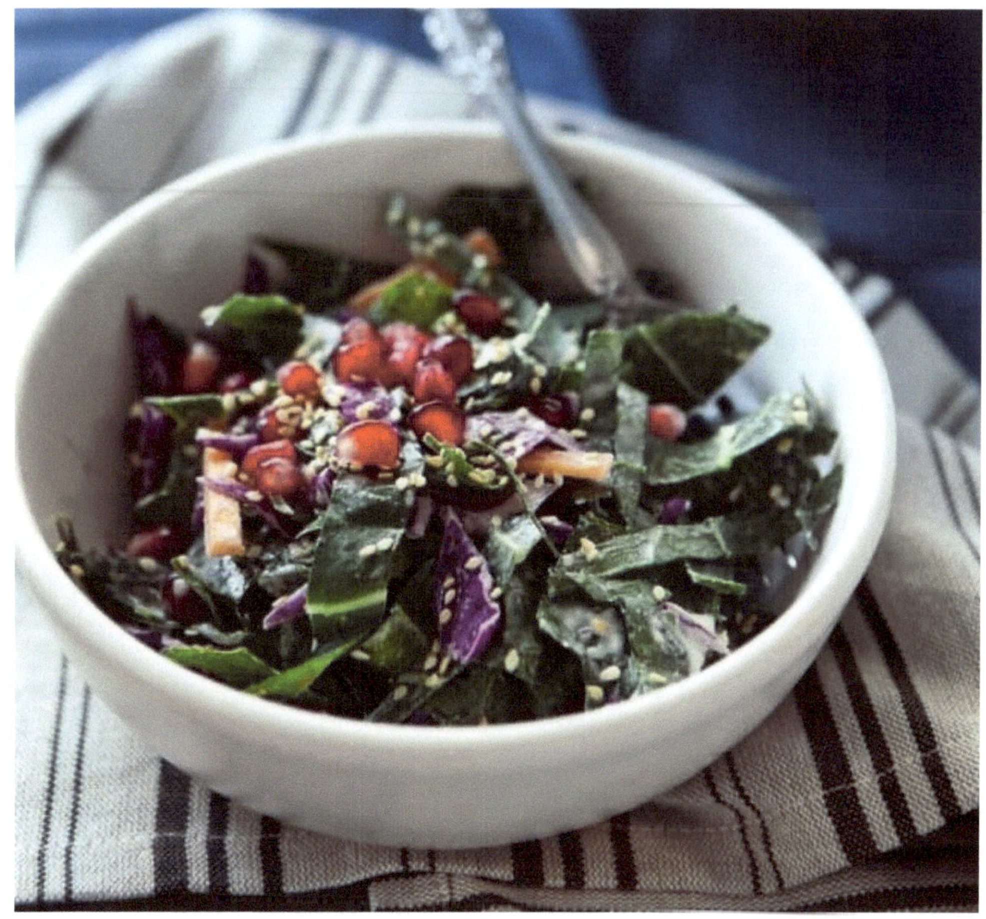

You'll love this version of salad with a dose of apple cider vinegar in the dressing.

Serves 6 to 8

Ingredients:

For the slaw:

- 1 bunch collard greens, rinsed and thinly sliced into 2-inch-long pieces
- 2 medium carrots, peeled and julienned
- 1 ripe red apple, cored and julienned
- 1/2 bunch flat-leaf Italian parsley, finely chopped
- 1/2 cup pomegranate seeds, plus more to top
- 1/2 small head red cabbage, finely shredded
- 3 green onions, thinly sliced
- 1/3 cup toasted sesame seeds
- Kosher salt and black pepper, to season

For the dressing:

- 1/4 cup tahini
- 1 heaping teaspoon Dijon mustard
- 1/4 cup apple cider vinegar
- 1 teaspoon honey
- Generous pinch of kosher salt

Instructions:

1. Combine all of the slaw ingredients into a very large salad bowl.
2. To make the dressing, whisk together the tahini, mustard, apple cider vinegar, honey, and salt until smooth and creamy. If the dressing seems clumpy or too thick to coat the greens well, add a little water, 1 teaspoon at a time.
3. Toss the salad with the dressing. Sprinkle extra pomegranate seeds on top and serve.

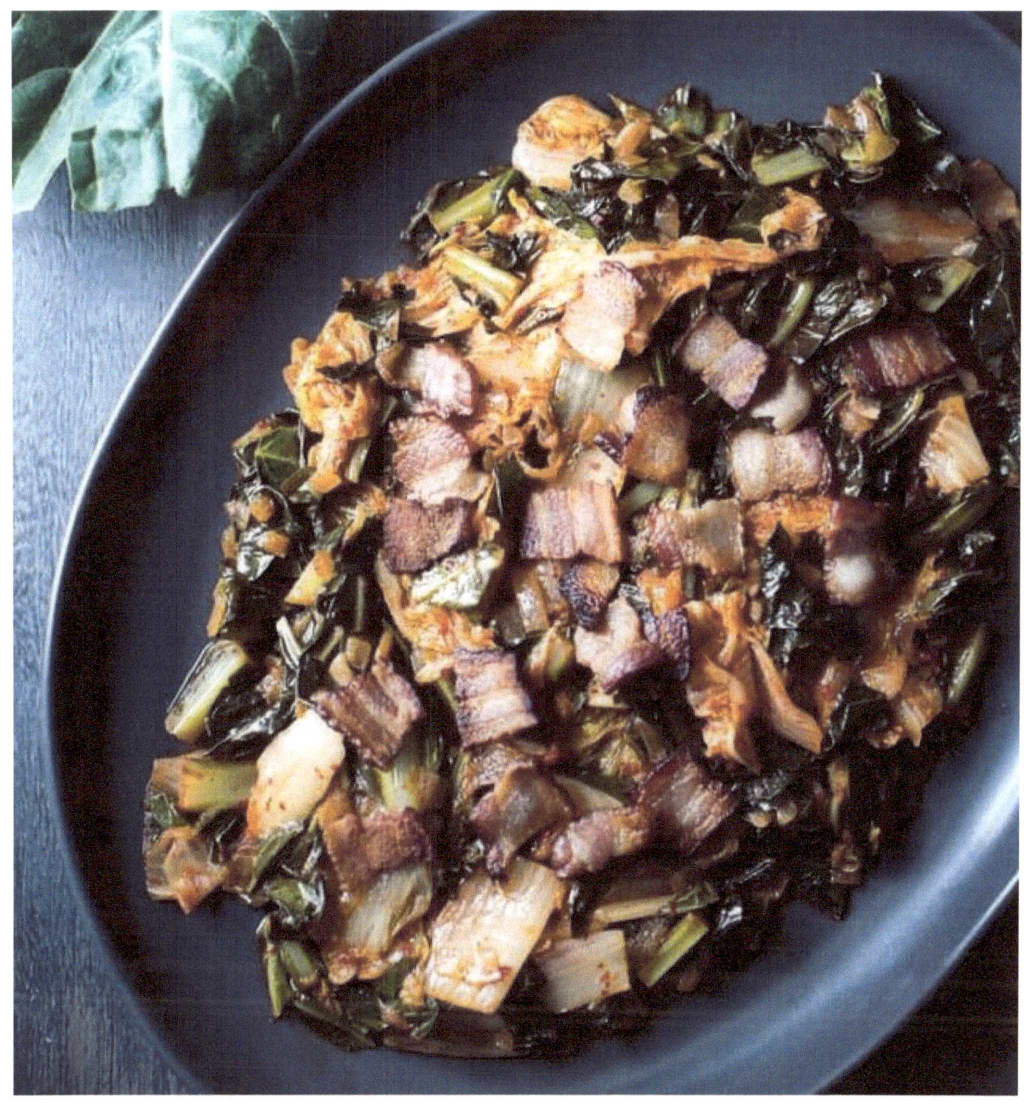

The apple cider vinegar here is used to deglaze the pan that the bacon.

Serves 4 to 6

Ingredients:

- 1 tablespoon olive oil
- 5 slices thick-cut bacon, cut into 1-inch pieces
- 1/2 medium sweet onion, peeled and diced
- 2 bunches collard greens
- 2 tablespoons apple cider vinegar
- 1 cup low-sodium chicken or vegetable broth
- 1 (14-ounce) jar kimchi
- Pinch of red pepper flakes (optional)

Instructions:

Cooking the bacon

1. Heat the oil in a very large skillet (not nonstick) over medium-high until it shimmers.
2. Add chopped bacon and cook until crisp around the edges, stirring occasionally with a wooden spoon.
3. Remove bacon to a paper towel-lined plate and set aside. With bacon grease still in the skillet, add onion and sauté until softened, translucent, and nearly caramelized, 8 to 10 minutes.

Preparing the collards

1. While the bacon and onion are cooking, stack a few collard leaves on a cutting board.
2. Cut off stems and cut leaves crosswise into long. 1-inch wide strips. Cut strips into approximate 2-inch pieces. Repeat with remaining collard leaves.
3. Place collards in a colander or salad spinner and rinse under running water; spin or shake dry to remove most of the water.
4. When onion is nearly caramelized, add collards, one handful at a time.
5. Heat and stir until collards begin to cook down, about 2 minutes, then add another handful of collards.
6. Repeat until all collards are added to the skillet.

Deglazing the pan

1. Push collards to one side of the skillet to expose the browned bits (the fond) on the bottom of the pan.
2. Add the apple cider vinegar and quickly stir up the fond.
3. Add broth, reduce heat to medium, and continue to cook collards, stirring occasionally, until almost all of the liquid is evaporated, 10 to 15 minutes.
4. Meanwhile, open the jar of kimchi over the sink since fermented foods have a tendency to bubble over when opened.
5. When the liquid in the skillet has nearly all evaporated (and what liquid remains has turned golden-brown and thickened), remove skillet from heat.
6. Add kimchi to ingredients in skillet and stir until well-mixed. If desired, stir in red pepper flakes.
7. Transfer collards-kimchi mixture to a serving dish and top with the crisp bacon pieces.
8. Serve warm.

About the Author

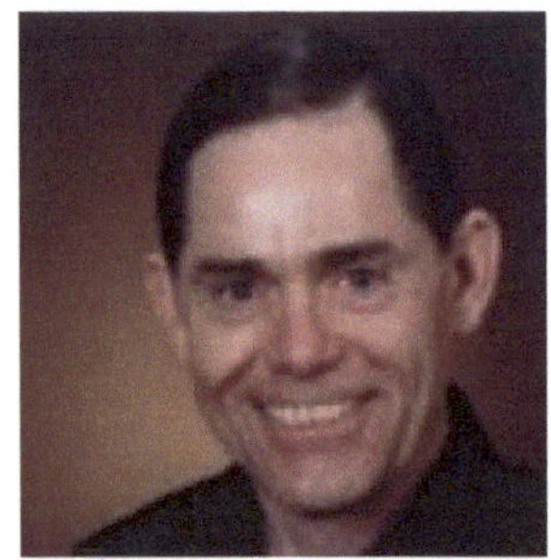

I have published numerous books on Amazon (both for Kindle and in paperback), along with other publishing platforms.

I'm proud to publish a broad range of books for readers interested in health and fitness — including books on Yoga, Weight Loss, Fitness, Lifestyle and Nutrition and much more. A complete list of our books can be found at https://www.amazon.com/Ron-Kness/e/B0072M6PYO.

Besides my own writing, I also ghostwrite ebooks, books, reports, articles, blogs and do Kindle conversions for clients on a variety of topics. Contact me for a quote at my website https://ronknesswriting.com.

Today my wife and I are retired from our careers and live in Gold Canyon, AZ. I now write as a retirement business where you'll find me happily sitting in my office typing away on my laptop as I work on my next book or ghostwriting project . . . that is if we are not traveling on a cruise ship - our new-found mode of travel.

www.ingramcontent.com/pod-product-compliance
Lightning Source LLC
Chambersburg PA
CBHW040047240726
48664CB00004B/1099